Workhouse nursing (annotated)

by Florence Nightingale

The accompanying account of the Improvements introduced by the Select Vestry of Liverpool into the Workhouse Hospital Wards under their control, may perhaps be interesting to you, and possibly might prove suggestive and serviceable, if similar improvements should be required in your district.

As the time and strength of the Lady Superintendent of the Nurses employed in the Workhouse Hospital are very fully occupied, enquiries or requests for further information should not be addressed to her, but to the Chairman of the Workhouse Committee of the Select Vestry (and of the Hospital Sub-Committee),

T. H. SATCHELL, Esq.
48, Lord Street,
Liverpool;

Or,

H. J. HAGGER, Esq.
Parish Offices,
Liverpool.

WORKHOUSE NURSING:

THE STORY OF A SUCCESSFUL EXPERIMENT.

The following pages contain a brief account of the experiment successfully tried by the Select Vestry of Liverpool (the guardians of the poor)—the introduction of trained Nurses into the male wards of the Workhouse Infirmary. That experiment having resulted so successfully as to induce the Vestry to extend the system to the remainder of the infirmary, it may be interesting to those who are concerned in the management of workhouses elsewhere to learn something of its history and progress. It is the writer's object to explain —

1. The grounds on which the Vestry were led to undertake the experiment, as stated in the preliminary report of Mr. Carr, the governor, and that of the sub-committee of the Vestry appointed to consider the proposed scheme; and the replies received to inquiries addressed by them to institutions and persons connected with the training and employment of skilled nurses in London and Liverpool, with letters on the subject from Miss Nightingale and Sir John McNeill.

2. The results of the experiment, so far as hitherto ascertained.

The Liverpool Vestry had previously made considerable efforts to improve the workhouse infirmaries. The medical men had been encouraged to make requisition for every material appliance that could facilitate the cure of the sick; and paid female officers were appointed at the rate of one to each 150 or 200 beds, to superintend the giving of medicines and stimulants, and so forth: but of course so small a number, even had they been trained nurses, could do no real nursing, and could exercise little supervision over the twenty drunken or unreliable[1] pauper nurses who were under the nominal direction of each paid officer. An appeal was made to the Vestry to consummate the good work they had thus partially commenced, and it was urged that Liverpool should assume the lead in the task of workhouse reform. The following considerations were submitted to the Select Vestry:—

"That Liverpool could commence this movement with great effect, and with the certainty that her example would be widely followed.

"That she had in times past taken a leading part in such reform. The introduction of the New Poor Law produced little change in Liverpool; so many of its wisest provisions were already in operation there, some of them for twenty or thirty years.

"That she had already established a system of attention to the sick poor in their own houses, which, if only by restoring heads of families to health and work, saved the parish many times the sum that it cost to private benevolence.

"That, lastly and especially, the proposed reform ought to commence in Liverpool, because in her workhouse the guardians had already, by their liberality, provided the sick with everything in the shape of diet and medical comforts that could conduce to recovery; and what was now wanting to give effect to their wise benevolence was, that their system should be administered and their intentions carried out by efficient and reliable nurses, in the stead of unreliable paupers."

The appeal further urged that—

"Successful efforts have been made in many directions to improve the nursing of the sick, and the workhouses must soon be the object of similar endeavours. Those poor sufferers whose disease is protracted and hopeless are refused admission into ordinary hospitals, and must come to the workhouse; and the mere duration of the illness is in such cases sufficient to reduce to poverty the most industrious, careful, and temperate—men who, while they could work, paid regularly their contribution to the poor-rate. Surely, these are entitled to at least as great care as that which sickness at once assures to the imprisoned felon, however criminal, for whom well-paid nurses are provided by the State.

"As to the other class of inmates of the workhouse infirmary—those whose ailments are curable—mere economy requires that the most efficient means should be taken to cure them as speedily as possible, so as to preserve them and their families from becoming paupers.

"Thus justice and expediency alike counsel the introduction into the workhouse of the best known system of nursing. Probably nothing which the skill and kindness of medical men can do, no food or physical appliances which the guardians can supply, no oversight or care which they, acting through pauper nurses, can bring to bear, are wanting in the Liverpool workhouse; but it is to be feared that much of this care, liberality, and thought fails of its object for want of a sufficient number of reliable and duly qualified nurses to carry out the instructions given, to administer food and medicine to the patients, to dress their wounds, and so forth."

This appeal was supported by two letters of Miss Nightingale and Sir John McNeill, G.C.B., President of the Board of Supervision (the Scotch Poor Law Board).

Letter from Miss Nightingale.

115, Park Street, W.
February 5, 1864.

My dear Sir,

I will not delay another day expressing how much I admire, and how deeply I sympathize with the Workhouse plan.

First let me say that Workhouse sick and Workhouse Infirmaries require quite as much care as (I had almost said more than) Hospital sick. There is an even greater work to be accomplished in Workhouse Infirmaries than in Hospitals.

In days long ago, when I visited in one of the largest London Workhouse Infirmaries, I became fully convinced of this.

How gladly would I have become the Matron of a Workhouse.

But of a Visitor's visit, the only result is to break the Visitor's heart. She sees how much could be done and cannot do it.

Liverpool is of all places the one to try this great Reform in. Its example is sure to be followed. It has an admirable body of Guardians; it is a thorough practical people; it has, or soon will have again, money.

Lord Russell once said (what is quite true), that the Poor Law was never meant to supersede private charity.

But whatever may be the difficulties about Pauperism, in two things most people agree—viz. that Workhouse sick ought to have the best practical nursing, as well as Hospital sick—and that a good wise Matron may save many of these from life-long pauperism, by first nursing them well, and then rousing them to exertion, and helping them to employment.

In such a scheme as is wisely proposed, there would be four elements.

1. The Guardians, one of whose functions is to check pauperism. They could not be expected to incur greater cost than at present, unless it is proved that it cures or saves life.

2. The Visiting or Managing Committee of the Guardians, whose authority must not (and need not) in any way be interfered with.

3. The Governor, the Medical Officer, and Chaplain.

4. (And under the Governor) the proposed Superintendent of Nurses and her nursing staff.

There is no reason why all these parts of the machine should not work together.

The funds are provided to pay the extra nursing for a time.

The difficulty is to find the Lady to govern it.

When appointed, she must be authorized—indeed appointed—by the Guardians. She must be their Officer; and must be invested by the Governor with authority to superintend her Nurses in conformity with regulations to be agreed upon.

So far, I see no more difficulty than there was in settling our relations as Nurses to the government officials in the Crimean War.

The cases are somewhat similar.

As to the funds, it is just possible that eventually the Guardians might take all the cost on themselves, as soon as they saw the great advantages and economy of good nursing.

If Liverpool succeeds, the system is quite sure to extend itself.

The Fever Hospital is one of the Workhouse Infirmaries. That is the place to shew what skilful nursing can do. The patients are not all paupers. How many families might be rescued from pauperism by saving the lives of their heads, and by helping the hard-working to more speedy convalescence!

Hopefully yours,
(Signed) FLORENCE NIGHTINGALE.

Extract from a letter from the Right Honourable Sir John McNeill, G.C.B., dated Granton House, Edinburgh, 28th Feb., 1864.

There can be no doubt, I think, that it would be a mistake to have pauper nurses mixed up with paid nurses, and I think I expressed that opinion when we conversed about those things. Paupers might, however, be employed to scrub and to do other menial work, under the orders of the paid nurses. If the paid nurses are to do much good they must have a recognised authority in their wards. Without authority there cannot be due responsibility, and things must get into confusion. A nurse carrying out the instructions of the medical officer must have authority to do so, and resistance to that authority must be treated as a breach of discipline.

To put this upon a right footing from the first, would be indispensable to success. The more a nurse does by influence, and kindly influence, the better; but dealing with the promiscuous inmates of a workhouse, the knowledge that there is authority in reserve to be exercised if necessary, prevents the necessity of resorting to it, and makes the patients duly appreciate the kindness which keeps it in reserve.

With regard to all such matters, a great deal will depend upon the good-will, the good sense, and good feeling of the Governor and Matron, but especially of the Governor. He can do much to promote or to mar the success of the experiment, and so can the medical men; but if they be men of sense and right feeling, they cannot fail to perceive how vast an addition to their own comfort the permanent establishment of such a system as you propose to introduce experimentally, must produce.

The position of a medical man dependent for the execution of his instructions upon nurses who are neither intelligent nor trustworthy, is very painful, and tends to deteriorate his own character, both as a man and as a practitioner, by rendering him callous to preventible suffering which he is denied the proper means of relieving, and by compelling him to forego the use of remedies which require intelligence and conscientious care in administering them. The house Governor, if he be a conscientious man, must be kept in continual anxiety about the conduct of ignorant, and often worthless pauper nurses in the hospital, and is driven at length to be satisfied with a low moral and intellectual standard in the nurses, and a corresponding standard of care and comfort in the hospital.

The Select Vestry took the subject into their serious consideration, and instituted most careful inquiries in various quarters. Among other steps, they called for a report on the probable operation of the proposed system from Mr. Carr, the Governor of the Workhouse. That report ran as follows: —
Extract from the Journal of the Governor of the Workhouse.

Liverpool, Thursday, April 14, 1864.

In compliance with the instructions of the Workhouse Committee, I have carefully considered the proposal made to the Committee by a Liverpool gentleman, on the subject of nursing the sick in the Workhouse Hospital, and beg in reference thereto to report —

That, practically, the proposal amounts to this—that there shall not be any pauper nurses in the hospital, but that there shall be appointed in lieu a staff of duly qualified paid nurses and servants, with a head superintendent, under whom the whole of the nursing of the sick shall be conducted on the best known principles.

This proposal rests its claim to favourable consideration on the presumption that the present system of nursing the sick in the Workhouse Hospital is defective. The Committee are aware what that system is. It may thus be briefly stated. Certain wards of the workhouse are set apart as hospital wards. They do not form an hospital worked as a whole, but are divided into five portions, each forming a distinct set of wards, in close proximity to the wards of the healthy paupers, and in five different parts of the workhouse. These five sets of wards I shall call the Workhouse Hospital. The hospital is divided into eleven sections. At the head of each section there is an intelligent paid superintendent nurse, and under each such superintendent nurse there is placed a staff of pauper nurses, with the aid of whom she is required to work her division, according to certain rules and regulations made and provided for that purpose. A copy of these rules is appended hereto; from which it will be seen that the burden of the responsibility of carrying out the orders of the medical officers, devolves upon the head nurses or superintendents of divisions. The pauper nurses clean up the wards, carry the food, and give general assistance to the superintendent—the duties of nursing in detail, that is to say, the bedside nursing, falling chiefly upon them. They are not permitted, however, to serve any patient with stimulants, beer, porter, or medicines requiring exactness or care; all such duties are discharged by the superintendent nurse. The proposal now made to the Committee, means that the paid staff shall be increased, so that the sick shall be cared for by responsible officers only, and not left, even partially, to the care of pauper nurses.

There is no doubt that pauper nurses are unreliable, inefficient, and many of them very worthless; and it is only by careful watching, and the utmost stringency of regulations, that they can be made serviceable in the hospital. No stringency of regulations, however, could guard against the most flagrant abuses, if these women were employed to discharge duties of trust, such as serving out the stimulants, &c. so that their services in attending upon the sick are limited and common-place. There is therefore, in my mind, no doubt, and I cannot see how any doubt can exist, that to remove these women, and appoint in their places women of character, trained as nurses, will tend to improve the position of the sick, and more rapidly restore many of them to health.

To displace these pauper women, however, involves a complete change in all the hospital arrangements, and suggests the difficulty of finding and keeping up a supply of suitable nurses to undertake the work at, as it would no doubt often happen, short notice. The Committee are aware, too, that owing to the fact that the paupers have hitherto been required to attend upon the sick, the accommodation for paid officers is very limited, and that the adoption of the proposal would render it necessary at once to provide additional rooms for the additional staff. The Committee are also aware that the Workhouse Hospital differs from other hospitals in this—that it forms a part only of a mixed establishment, and that there are great difficulties to be overcome in completely cutting off every connexion or species of intercourse between the hospital departments and the healthy inmates, without which the scheme under consideration could hardly succeed. If any good is to result from the adoption of this proposal, the sick should be placed absolutely and entirely in the hands of a paid staff, without the assistance, in any form, of any one of the pauper inmates. Cut off the hospital department from the healthy wards; and do not, under any pretext, suffer communication between the sick and the healthy, and you strike at the root of every species of workhouse abuse; but if, under any pretext, you suffer a large number of healthy paupers to pass daily into the sick departments, as they now do, the adoption of the proposal will effect little good.

But the question has to be still further investigated on the ground of expense; and it has to be decided the number, pay, allowances, and accommodation of the necessary staff to work it out. Now, although I entertain very strong opinions as to the undesirability of employing paupers to discharge responsible duties of any kind, because to do so destroys the value of the workhouse test, and tends to reconcile them to pauperism; and although I view the particular work of nurse-tending as the very worst kind of work for paupers, inasmuch as, while so employed, they are better fed, have more freedom of action than they otherwise would, and can make their places emolumental—thereby holding out a positive inducement to pauperism; and although I have no doubt that the displacement of these women would be followed by the immediate application for discharges by a large per-centage of them; and although, at this moment, many other weighty considerations press upon me in favour of the immediate adoption of the proposal under consideration, I feel unwilling, in view of the difficulties to be overcome, some of which I have indicated, to incur the weighty responsibility of recommending such a course on my own unaided judgment. I have abstained, therefore, from taking up the question of expense, &c. but take the liberty respectfully to suggest, that a sub-committee be appointed to report upon the whole question in all its details. It shall be my anxious desire and pleasure to assist the labours of such sub-committee by every means in my power.

According to the recommendation of Mr. Carr, a Sub-Committee was appointed, consisting of men of great experience in parochial business, who went up to London, and had interviews with the medical and other officers of the two metropolitan hospitals where nursing has been brought to the greatest perfection—St. Thomas's and King's College Hospitals. Finding that some of these gentlemen wished for more information respecting the Workhouse Hospital system before they would venture to express decided opinions as to the economical results of the proposed reform, the Liverpool Visitors drew up a statement on several points affecting this question, with written inquiries, to which answers were returned, verbally or in writing, by the gentlemen consulted. This statement, with the replies which it elicited, is here given at length:—[2]

STATEMENT AND QUESTIONS OF THE LIVERPOOL SUB-COMMITTEE.

The population of the Parish of Liverpool is about 270,000.

The expenditure from the poor's-rate in and about the relief of the poor is about 100,000l. per annum.

Of this about 40,000l. is distributed in out-door relief as money and bread. (Of course sickness is one great cause of persons seeking relief, though to what extent this cause operates, even directly, I cannot on so short a notice ascertain or even estimate.)

The expenses (direct) of treating the out-door sick are:—

Salaries of Medical Officers, &c. £1,800
Medicines, &c. 1,378
 £3,178

The cost of maintaining the Workhouse Hospital may be estimated as follows:—

Maintenance of Patients £9,700
Salaries of Medical Officers 485
Medicines, &c 1,050
£11,235

The Hospital contains accommodation for over 1,000 patients, and has often 1,000 in it. The cases at present are:—

Medical 485
Surgical 345

Fever 120

Smallpox 20

The weekly discharges are from twenty to thirty per cent, of the whole number in the hospital.[3]

The present workhouse staff consists of fourteen paid officers (who are superintendents, but not trained nurses), and about 150 paupers acting as nurses, but not paid. It has been proposed to add a trained hospital matron and trained nurses, such as those trained in the Nightingale School, and assistant nurses, so as to give one trained day-nurse and one paid assistant to about every three pauper nurses, and a trained night-nurse on every flat; it is further proposed to pay the paupers who act as nurses, wages. The cost of this would be about 2,000l. per annum.

Does your experience of hospitals lead you to believe that the cost of this improved system would be "in part," "wholly," or "more than" repaid to the ratepayers by curing people more quickly, by curing those who otherwise might have become chronic cases, and by enabling those to resume their work who must otherwise have remained or died, and by thus diminishing the duration or amount of that part of pauperism which is the result of sickness?

REPLIES OF PHYSICIANS, &c. OF ST. THOMAS'S HOSPITAL.

1. Reply of R. H. Goolden, Esq., M.D.

"I have no doubt but that the plan suggested, if properly carried out, would be in the end a saving to the ratepayers, the restoration to health relieving the parish of constant burdens."

2. Reply of John Simon, Esq.

"I do not feel myself competent to measure at all exactly what might be the pecuniary result of the proposed system. But in my opinion the substitution of skilled for unskilled attendance would be of great advantage to the sick, and would of course tend to diminish that part of the pauperism which results from sickness."

3. Reply of Sydney Jones, Esq., M.D.

"In my opinion the improved system of nursing recommended would amply repay the expense incurred."

4. Reply of J. S. Bristowe, Esq., M.D.

"I believe that the introduction of paid nurses into the Liverpool Workhouse Infirmary would be of inestimable benefit to the sick poor received into the institution, and would thus amply justify the expense which it is proposed to incur. I also think it very probable that the cost of nursing would be repaid in many other ways to the ratepayers."

5. Reply of Edward Clapton, Esq., M.D.

"I believe it would be quite repaid."

REPLIES FROM THE PHYSICIANS, &c. OF KING'S COLLEGE HOSPITAL.

1. Reply of Henry Smith, Esq, Assistant Surgeon.

"I believe, from a long experience of hospitals and other institutions, that the cost of an improved system of nursing as proposed for the Liverpool Workhouse Hospital would certainly be 'in part ' repaid by restoring the patients to health more quickly."

2. Copy of a Letter from Miss Jones, Lady Superintendent of St, John's House Nursing Schools, and Matron of Kings College Hospital.

King's College Hospital, May 4, 1864.

Dear Sir,

The inclosed paper was sent to me yesterday, with the request that I would obtain from some of the medical staff of this Hospital answers to the question proposed at the end of the paper, in order to enable the Vestry in some degree to judge whether that body would be justified, or otherwise, in sanctioning the introduction to their Workhouse Hospital of an improved system of nursing the sick, at the probable annual money cost named in the inclosed paper.

I have accordingly submitted the paper to as many of the medical staff as I could see in the short time.

I inclose a note from Mr. Henry Smith, one of the surgeons, who has had considerable experience as to the loss and gain of good and bad nursing.

Dr. Wm. O. Priestly, the Physician Accoucheur to this Hospital, formerly of Middlesex Hospital, had not time during his visit to do more than read the paper and give me a verbal answer. He said, "I have no hesitation in saying that the saving would be certain and great."

The Assistant Physician Accoucheur, who has until last week had charge of the medical patients here, as House Physician (Mr. H. L. Kempthorne), says, "The value of trained efficient nursing cannot be overrated in the management of acute diseases, and especially fevers, and would speak for itself in the saving of life, humanly speaking.

"In chronic cases, the eye of the trained nurse would soon detect the malingerer, and thus save the parish the expense of maintaining one who could well keep himself.

"In the prevention and amelioration of disease this plan would soon show its importance in the effects of cleanliness, ventilation, and other points carried out systematically and intelligently.

"The moral influence of the trained nurses by precept and example must in time diffuse itself through the medium of the pauper nurses to the paupers in hospital, the workhouse, and thence to the parish at large."

I regret my inability to obtain fuller testimony to-day, but professional men are busy, and their visits to the hospital only on stated days.

If I can be of further use in any way, pray command me.

I am. Sir,
Very faithfully yours,
(Signed) M.J.
Superintendent of St. John's.

After collecting and considering all the information within their reach, the Sub-Committee reported as follows:—

The Sub-Committee appointed on the 14th ultimo to consider and report as to a suggested alteration in the Staff of the Workhouse Hospital, report,

That the superiority, as nurses, of trained, experienced, and responsible women to the pauper women upon whom, under the present system, the actual nursing of the sick inmates of the workhouse devolves, is so apparent, that they conceive it to be unnecessary to offer any further observations upon this part of the subject. The points which have mainly occupied your Committee's attention are the following:—
1.The cost of introducing a staff of trained nurses into the Workhouse Hospital, or any portion thereof.
2.The practicability of providing sufficient accommodation in the Workhouse for such an increase of officers.

3.The supply of trained nurses.

1. Your Committee are of opinion that the substitution throughout the Workhouse Hospital of trained nurses, for the present pauper nurses, would involve a direct expenditure of from 2,000l. to 2,500l. per annum. Should it be decided, in the first instance, to introduce the nurses into the male hospital only, it is probable that a sum of 800l. per annum would be found sufficient for the purpose. Evidence has been laid before the Committee to show that in those hospitals where the improved system of nursing has been introduced, the increased cost thereof has been more than compensated for by the saving, from the reduction of the time during which the patients are under treatment — the effect, as is alleged, of good and efficient nursing. Whilst your Committee admit the force of the argument, that if this be so in the case of hospitals, where the sick only are burdens upon the funds of the institution, much more must it be so in the case of the parish, where, as often happens, the whole family are chargeable upon the rates in consequence of the sickness of its head; they think it necessary to point out that one great difference between the workhouse hospital and an ordinary infirmary consists in this, that while in the latter (as a rule) none but acute and supposed curable cases are admitted, the former is, in many cases, the refuge of those who, as incurables, cannot gain admittance to other asylums. There can, however, be no doubt that the saving resulting from the rapidity and completeness of the cures effected by good nursing, will be a considerable set-off against the increased cost of the nursing staff; though your Committee can offer no decided opinion as to the probable extent of the saving so effected.

2. Your Committee believe that accommodation equal at least, if not superior, to that afforded to the nurses in the London hospitals, can be provided in the Workhouse at a moderate outlay. It is estimated that, for the male hospital, a sum of from 400l. to 500l, would suffice to provide the rooms and to furnish them.

3. With reference to the supply of suitable nurses, your Committee have to

report that, as the authorities of the Nightingale Training School for nurses have offered to render to the Select Vestry all the assistance in their power in obtaining trained nurses, no great difficulty on this point need be apprehended.

Were your Committee as sanguine as some of the hospital authorities whom they have consulted, as to the happy results to be expected from the introduction of trained nurses into the Workhouse, they would at once, with the utmost confidence, recommend that the whole of the hospital should, at the cost of the parish, be supplied with this class of officers; but, looking upon it as they do, as an experiment (at least in its economical results), they unanimously recommend that the system should, in the first instance, be tried in the male hospital

J. W. CROPPER, Chairman.

May 5, 1864.

The report of the Sub-Conimittee met with the approval of the Vestry. Some delay in the adoption of its recommendations was caused by a severe outbreak of fever in the town, which for the time absorbed all the resources of the Vestry and its officers. But on the 18th of May, 1865, a Lady Superintendent who had received a thorough training at Kaiserswerth and St. Thomas's, twelve Nightingale nurses from St. Thomas's, eighteen probationers, and fifty-two of the old pauper nurses were placed in charge of the patients in the male wards of the Workhouse Infirmary. By the judicious management of Mr. Carr, the most admirable arrangements were made for the accommodation of the nurses. Each superior nurse had a little room to herself, and the ex-pauper nurses were entirely separated from the other inmates of the Workhouse. It was hoped that by taking the best of the able-bodied inmates, separating them from the other paupers, and paying them small wages (say 5l. a year) they might be made available as assistant nurses, and that many of them might be elevated into independence and usefulness. It will be seen from the foregoing report of the Governor (p. 10), that he always distrusted this part of the plan adopted; and after the system had been at work a year, this attempt to utilize pauper nurses in a workhouse hospital was found to have utterly failed. It was proved that in a town like Liverpool, with very few exceptions, those able-bodied women only become inmates of the Workhouse who are either tainted in character, or are exceptionally ill-educated and inefficient. The experiment, however, was not wholly useless. It conclusively established two facts: that such women are utterly unfit to be trusted as nurses; and that their employment in that capacity does not effect all the saving that might be supposed. It might be thought that the choice lay between such employment and maintaining the pauper in idleness, while paying a nurse in her stead. But it was found—as the Governor had always predicted—that when sent back from the hospital to the able-bodied wards, nearly the whole of these women left the Workhouse, and relieved the parish from the charge of their maintenance. Many of these women, when employed as nurses, remain in the Workhouse for the sake of what they can pick up or extort. And moreover, when they left it, the training they had received, such as it was, rendered them more intelligent, and perhaps not more unreliable nurses than those usually employed by the poor. It is not unlikely that in country places the unfitness of able-bodied paupers to become assistant nurses may be far less than it has been found to be in a great seaport town like Liverpool. They may probably be less universally tainted in character, and after a year or two of employment as under-nurses they may be able to maintain themselves in that capacity out-of-doors, thus not only relieving the parish of their own maintenance, but assisting to diminish sickness and pauperism among their neighbours. The point is one which must be left to local knowledge and experience. It might be well, however, not to promise them payment till after some length of probationary service. It was always after pay-day that the ex-pauper nurses were most liable to get drunk and misbehave.[4] With the exception of the failure of the nurses taken from the pauper class, the first year's trial was sufficiently successful to induce a continuance of the experiment. It was impossible, however, to judge the result by statistics. None that were available could be considered as an evidence of success or failure, for several reasons. The season was very unhealthy, and to relieve the pressure on the space and resources of the hospital, steps were taken to treat slight cases outside, as will be seen from the following extract from the Minutes of the Finance Committee, 24th November, 1865:—

"The district medical officers, Dr. Gee, Mr. Barnes, and the Governor of the workhouse being in attendance, pursuant to resolution of the Workhouse Committee at its meeting yesterday, the practicability of limiting the admissions to the Workhouse Hospital was considered, and the district medical officers were requested to co-operate with the relieving officers in limiting such admissions to those cases that cannot be properly treated outside the Workhouse."

The endeavour to limit the admissions to serious cases would of course affect the returns, both as regards the time taken in curing, and the proportion of deaths. Even had there been no exceptional disturbing element, there is a defect in the statistics of workhouse hospitals which affects all inferences from them, in the absence of any careful classified list of cases kept by the medical officers, such as might fairly enable one to form a judgment from mere statistical tables. These, then, are not reliable as means of judgment, unless extending over a long period. The character of seasons, and nature of cases admitted, varies so much from year to year as to invalidate any deductions, unless founded on plete and minutely kept medical records. The following extracts, however, from the reports of the Governor, and the surgical and medical officers of the Workhouse, bear decisive witness to the value of the "new system," especially as contrasted with the "old system," which in 1865-66 still prevailed in the female wards. All these reports bear emphatic testimony to the merits and devotion of the Lady Superintendent and her staff. The medical men, it is noteworthy, speak strongly of the better discipline and far greater obedience to their orders observable where the trained nurses are employed—a point the more important because it is that on which, before experience has reassured them, medical and other authorities have often been most doubtful.

From the Report of the Governor.

Thursday, May 10, 1866.

The main feature in the new system of nursing consists in the superseding of pauper nurses, and appointing in their places competent trained nurses from the Nightingale School. These latter to have the assistance of "probationary nurses," or in other words, women of intelligence and of good character desirous of entering upon the duties of nursing the sick as a profession. A third class was also created, designated "Assistants." These were selected from the old pauper nurses, and it was decided that they should be paid, clothed, and receive rations equal in quality and quantity to those issued to the officers of the workhouse. The nurses, probationers, and assistants were placed under the control of a "Lady Superintendent," who was empowered to employ them in the manner to her seeming best for the proper care of the sick.

The Committee will be prepared to hear that the change was immediately followed by the most marked improvement in every respect. The most casual observer could not avoid perceiving it. This applies not only to the state of the wards, the care of the sick, but is particularly observable in the demeanour of the patients, upon whom the humanizing influences of a body of women of character, devotedly discharging their duties, has produced evident fruits.

The question has often been asked whether the "new system is likely to succeed?" The "old system" meant nothing more than this, that old, ignorant, and unreliable pauper women, many of whom were of doubtful character, were entrusted with the discharge, without pay, of responsible duties. These have been displaced, and active, intelligent, reliable women, trained and skilled as nurses, with good characters and pay, have been appointed to supersede them. It would be a great discredit if these latter did not discharge their duties incomparably better than the former could do. That they do so I am happy to be in a position to testify.

In the opening paragraph of this report it is stated that "assistant nurses" were appointed and placed upon pay from the ranks of the paupers. This I was always opposed to. Their employment has resulted in complete failure, as the following figures will prove. The total number appointed to this date is 141. Of these sixty-seven have been dismissed through drunkenness and other misconduct, and sixteen have resigned; while it is positively true that there is not one of the whole number to whom I could entrust the duties of serving out wine or other stimulants, or, in fact, any duty requiring the exercise of integrity.

The experience of the past year renders it certain that the Poor Law, as now existing, offers no impediments to the successful working out of the most complete scheme for the efficient nursing of the sick, in the manner advocated by the best friends of hospital nursing.

(Signed) GEO. CARR.

From the Report of Robert Gee, Esq. M.D. Physician to the Workhouse Hospital.
5, Abercromby Square, Liverpool,

May 10, 1866.

Sir,

In the medical wards of a general hospital the cases vary so much in nature and degree from year to year, as to render it impossible to give a reliable statistical comparison of the value of a paid as distinguished from an unpaid staff of nurses. I am, therefore, necessarily compelled to report in general terms on the nursing of the last ten months in the male medical wards; premising that what I say in approbation of the new system, and the new staff of nurses must not be construed as an unfavourable reflection on the whole of the previous staff. The paid superintending nurses of departments, and a few of the unpaid pauper nurses, deserve great credit for their conduct, though their qualifications for the service were decidedly inferior to those of the trained "Nightingale" staff.

With regard to the latter I can cordially bear testimony to their ability, and to their unwearied and uniformly kind attention to the patients under their charge. As to their nursing in its specific sense, I may state my belief that in every case my directions and those of the House Surgeons have been rigidly carried out. The medicines, stimulants, &c. &c. have been carefully administered, and the other numerous but less agreeable duties have been faithfully and efficiently attended to. Under their charge I have perceived a marked improvement in the demeanour of the patients—in fact, the discipline of the wards is completely changed. There has been no disorder or irregularity, but a sense of comfort, order, and quiet pervades the whole department. I believe further, that every patient leaving the wards has been more or less morally elevated during his location there.

From the report of J. H. Barnes, Esq., Surgeon.

March 21, 1866.

Since my connection with the hospital last August we have had somewhat approaching a hundred operations, many of them of a serious and dangerous character, requiring not only prompt assistance at the time, but most persevering attention night and day for a long time after. Almost all these operations have been in the male hospital, and I have no hesitation in saying that what success has attended them has been greatly owing to the most efficient assistance rendered by the trained nurses; and from my experience of the assistance received from the pauper nurses, in the few cases of operation performed in the female hospital, I should feel great diffidence in undertaking on that side such operations as I have had on the other side: indeed on one or two occasions the pauper nurses ran away, and when induced to assist were so nervous and frightened as to be of little service.

Without any wish to speak harshly of the unpaid nurses employed on the female side of the hospital (who, I believe, strive to do their best, more especially since a feeling of emulation has been set up by the introduction of the paid trained nurses, of whom they are jealous), I am compelled to state my conviction that on that side my directions are not carried out with that necessary promptitude and skill that they are on the other side, and that in all I do there I feel as if I were working with blunted instruments. There is no want of inclination, but simply a want of ability. That integrity of disposition, promptitude of action, tact in manipulation, gentleness of demeanour and kindly consideration necessary to make a nurse are not found, or to be found in the inmates of a workhouse, and no amount of education can work out of them what never was in them. Almost always obtuse, and too often unprincipled, as a class they are thoroughly unreliable and quite unfitted to take charge of the sick and helpless, or the stimulants necessary for them. On this last point I have been informed by a former resident surgeon that he has known the pauper nurses appropriate the patient's stimulants, or withhold giving to a dying patient that ordered for him, that they might take it themselves after his death. It is difficult to bring home and prove these things, and I do not wish to say they now occur, but if we wish to put such conduct out of the region of possibility it can only be done by the employment of persons superior to the temptation so to act.

Persons of one class, as a rule, favour their own class, and there is a far better chance of double-dealers being detected when under the observation and care of a trained nurse, than when under the care of one of themselves. That such is the case my own experience testifies.

As far, therefore, as my experience extends of the system of trained nurses, whether regarding the saving of life, the restoration to health, or the relief of the suffering, it has been an undoubted success.

These reports were duly considered by the authorities; and after some discussion, it was resolved entirely to discontinue, in the male hospital ward, the employment of paupers as assistant nurses, and to substitute an additional number of probationers. A Sub-Committee of the Workhouse

Committee was appointed to superintend and report upon the working of the system. These gentlemen devoted much time and attention to the subject, and at the close of the year undertook a minute inquiry into the operation of the old and new systems; examining personally the various officers of the Workhouse, from the Governor down to the pauper nurses in the female wards. Increased experience brought out in a yet stronger light the superior advantages of the employment of trained nurses. The very able, clear, and conclusive report of the Sub-Committee leaves little more to be said on the subject. It determined the Vestry to adopt the system in permanence, and to extend it to the whole of the Workhouse Infirmary, a year before the period fixed for the trial of the experiment had expired. It will be seen that the report of the second year's experience has a peculiar value, as bearing on the question whether, or how far, women may be competent to undertake one of the most delicate and difficult kinds of feminine work—one requiring special knowledge as well as special habits of punctual regularity, obedience, and thoughtfulness—without receiving any special training or education for such a duty. If the reforms about to be introduced into the pauper hospitals in London and elsewhere are not to end in failure and disappointment, provision must be made for training the nurses to be employed there, either before they enter the hospitals or within them. The report of the Sub-Committee of Superintendence is as follows:—

The Special Committee on Nursing, pursuant to resolution of the Workhouse Committee of the 7th of March instant, report,

That the Men's Hospital (exclusive of fever patients) is at present exclusively nursed by skilled, i. e. specially trained nurses and paid assistants, who are themselves undergoing training as nurses; the staff consisting of the Superintendent, nine of the nurses originally sent from the Nightingale School, five nurses who have been trained in the Workhouse, and fifteen probationary or assistant nurses.

Of the character of the nursing in this portion of the Workhouse, your Committee have heard but one opinion. The Governor and the Medical

Officers concur in speaking of it in terms of the highest praise, and throughout the whole period during which the Committee have superintended it, no single circumstance has come to their knowledge calculated to make them speak of it otherwise than in terms of approval.

The nursing of the women's wards continues to be done by paupers under the superintendence of paid officers. The superintendence of these officers is of necessity very imperfect, as not only has each charge of from 150 to 200 patients, but these patients are located in several rooms, each ward containing about twenty patients. The only portion of the nursing, properly so called, which these officers undertake, is the administration of stimulants and in some exceptional cases of medicine. The bulk of it, as the giving of medicine, the dressing of wounds, the distribution of food, is left to be done by paupers. So much has from time to time been said of the untrustworthiness of pauper nurses, of the evils resulting to those patients who are placed exclusively under them, of the mischievous consequences upon the discipline of the Workhouse of a large number of petty offices being filled by able-bodied women, that your Committee believe they rightly interpret the feeling of the Select Vestry, as they undoubtedly do that of the general public, in supposing that the actual nursing of the sick in the Liverpool Workhouse can no longer be left in the hands of pauper nurses.

Starting from this point, your Committee considered that they had principally to inquire what sort of nursing can be most advantageously substituted for that of nursing by paupers. Two courses only appeared to be open to them— either to increase the number of paid officers, giving to each such a number of patients as she could reasonably be expected to look after, and treating each as an independent officer; or to extend over the whole hospital the system now in existence in the men's wards. Your Committee were much aided in forming a judgment upon this point, by what has taken place during the last few months in the fever hospital.

Here, originally, the paid attendants were in precisely the same position, with precisely similar duties as the paid officers in the women's hospital; but the number of patients rapidly diminishing, and no corresponding reduction taking place in the number of officers, the staff was so large that Dr. Gee felt able to call upon the officers to act as nurses. The result was what might have been anticipated, that although an improvement upon the old system of nursing by paupers was perceptible, the state of the nursing was still far short of the standard reached in the men's wards.

The officers were told to nurse, and they did their best, but never having themselves been taught, their attempts in a great measure failed; they were paid and retained as nurses, without being efficient nurses.

Committee therefore recommend that as soon as the requisite number of trained nurses can be procured, the nursing in the women's hospital, and afterwards in the fever hospital, be placed in the hands of trained and skilled nurses, acting under the direction and control of Miss Jones, the present Superintendent. The expenses (beyond the item of wages) attendant upon the necessary increase in the number of nurses will not be great, as all that will be necessary will be to convert two of the rooms now used for sick boys into sleeping apartments for the nurses. In making this recommendation, the Committee are glad to know that they are fortified by the unanimous opinion of the Governor and the Medical Officers of the Workhouse.

Your Committee are bound to add that they can produce no statistics shewing that the nursing in the men's hospital has been of any economical advantage to the Parish; but as it needs no argument to prove that the cheapest course that can be taken with a sick pauper is to cure him as quickly as possible; as it is evident that the care and attention of a skilled nurse must tend to a more speedy recovery; as the order and discipline of a well-regulated ward is more distasteful to many of the more worthless inmates, than the laxer management of a room in the hands of a pauper nurse; and as the abolition of a large number of petty offices for able-bodied paupers must lead to many of them leaving the Workhouse, there are strong grounds for hoping that the economical results of the change cannot but be beneficial.

With regard to the future, your Committee recommend that the Department of Nursing should be placed under the direction of a small committee of your body, and that all changes in the staff should be made only by them. From information they have received, your Committee have reason to believe that if, after the Workhouse is supplied with Nurses, the two classes of nurses, i.e. trained nurses and probationers, be maintained, the cost of the Department may be considerably lessened by training nurses for other hospitals; the cost of the probationers being either paid for by a Government grant, or by the bodies for whom the nurses may be trained.

THOMAS H. SATCHELL,

RICHARD BRIGHT,

THOMAS OWEN.

March 15, 1867.

This report was unanimously adopted by the Workhouse Committee and by the Vestry; and already the new system has been extended to the Female Wards. It is in contemplation to extend it also to the Fever Hospital, as soon as a sufficient number of suitable nurses shall have been trained.

It will be observed that the report contemplates the training of probationers for other Workhouse Infirmaries. And it is, indeed, to be hoped that in this and other ways the Liverpool Workhouse Hospital may serve as a normal school, from which the system there adopted may spread. The special expenses of such a school would naturally be borne by the parishes which profited by its services in educating nurses for them, or by the Government. But this point is one which, as yet, has hardly demanded practical consideration.

The experiment whose results have been recorded, could hardly have been tried at all—certainly could not have achieved such rapid success—had it not been for the powerful and liberal assistance of Miss Nightingale, and the Trustees of the Nightingale Fund. Feeling how very important was the extension of the system of superior professional nursing, now gradually gaining ground in general hospitals, to workhouses, they sent, to assist in the initial experiment made in this direction, a lady superintendent and twelve superior nurses—a very expensive and quite invaluable contribution. To the Liverpool Vestry and its officers belongs the credit of having overcome all the difficulties, and persevered in spite of all the discouraging incidents, which necessarily attended an attempt to introduce a new system of management into such an institution as a Workhouse Hospital, combining as it does two subjects so different in their aspects and conditions of treatment, so difficult to deal with together, as pauperism and sickness. Of the Lady Superintendent I shall say little. When a lady leaves a happy home, and goes through a long and laborious course of training to fit herself for such a situation, purely because, feeling that she possessed the capacity for nursing, and the requisite health, energy, strength, and spirits, she desired to devote such powers to the service of those who stood most in need of them, human praise or criticism of her choice is out of place. One of the incidental results of her exertions has to her, no doubt, been even a higher reward than that improvement in the condition of the sick, in their progress towards recovery, and their material comfort, which has been the direct object of her labours. The improvement in the tone and behaviour of the patients has been wonderful. Many of the inmates of a pauper hospital are persons of the worst character, and its wards, under the control of pauper nurses, often present scenes so disgusting that the respectable poor shrink from them with utter abhorrence, and after once becoming acquainted with them, will often rather die than return thither. When the trained nurses were first introduced, the most offensive language was frequently heard in the wards; and the Lady Superintendent has repeatedly been obliged to call upon the Governor two or three times during one Sunday to use his authority to put a stop to actual fighting. Now, though his support is always promptly rendered, she is rarely compelled to apply for it; the feeling of the wards promptly suppresses all offensive language or unseemly behaviour in the presence of the nurses. The following letter from Sir H. Verney, Chairman of the Nightingale Committee, serves to illustrate the influence of the nurses upon the conduct of the patients; he came down to Liverpool to inspect the Hospital, and ascertain the progress of the work:—

Liverpool, October 3, 1866.

My dear Sir,

By the kindness of Mr. Carr I have paid a visit to the Workhouse, and have been greatly interested by remarking the change among the male pauper sick, effected since I was here about two years since. I conclude that this is owing to the nursing by a class of females so entirely different to those who nursed the male paupers at that time, and who still nurse the female sick. I have always seen that the influence of respectable and well-educated females over the most debased men is very striking. Men of that character, accustomed to intercourse with only degraded women, feel the restraining and humanizing power of virtuous and well-mannered females. They have never been admitted into intercourse with such before, and they are most beneficially affected by it. I have been told that the police officers, who sometimes come to the Workhouse on business, and who see the sick paupers, are much astonished. They see the men whom they have known as the very worst characters, conducting themselves with propriety and decency, and giving no cause of complaint.

I am sure that the Workhouse Committee must rejoice and feel thankful that there is such a change in the condition of the poor creatures brought under their rule.

Miss Jones, and her nurses and probationers, must have had much difficulty at first—indeed their work is still very trying; but the improved demeanour of the men must be highly gratifying and encouraging to them. I walked through the female sick wards; they were clean and sweet, but I could not help contrasting the pauper nurses who attended them, with the intelligent-looking respectable attendants of the men.

I thank you for the note of introduction which procured admission for me, and

I am,
  Yours very faithfully,
  HARRY VERNEY.

Such, and so entirely satisfactory to the Guardians, were the results of the experiment of nursing by trained nurses, as tried for two years in the Male Wards of the Liverpool Workhouse Infirmary. It is in order to render those results, the experience acquired in this initiatory attempt, available for the assistance and encouragement of others, that they have been thus briefly recorded. Much more might have been said; but what is here set down is sufficient to explain all that practical men would wish to know, and it would be presumption to waste the time of such men with comments and inferences which they are perfectly able to make for themselves.

One suggestion, in conclusion, I may be permitted to offer. In all unions or parishes where additional accommodation may be required, whether for patients or for healthy paupers, it is eminently desirable that in providing it regard should be had to the entire separation, at once or at a future time, of the sick and infirm from the able-bodied, as will be the case, at least partially, under the new régime introduced in the Metropolis by Mr. Gathorne Hardy's Bill. Miss Nightingale has from the first held and expressed a strong opinion in favour of the separation of the hospital and workhouse administrations. The Governor of the Liverpool Workhouse, Mr. Carr, expressed himself decidedly in the same sense; and the Chairman of the Workhouse Committee and of the Sub-Committee appointed to superintend the Hospital, has been induced by practical experience warmly to advocate the absolute separation of the Workhouse and the Infirmary. So large a proportion of the able-bodied inmates of the workhouse are drunken, lazy, and vicious, that, if the poor-law relief is not to become a temptation and an injury to the honest and struggling poor, the discipline must be almost of a penal character. The paramount object must be to make the workhouse, if not absolutely unpleasant, less agreeable than the condition of laborious and striving poverty. On the other hand, in a hospital the paramount and almost the only object is to promote recovery and to mitigate suffering; all other considerations yield to this, and consequently the treatment must necessarily be liberal in spirit and indulgent in fact. The modes of treatment necessary for the good management of the hospital patient and of the able-bodied pauper, respectively, are distinct—almost opposite: the infirmary and the workhouse must be controlled on divergent, and even contrary principles; and by bringing the two together under one roof and one administration, they injure each other. The indulgence of the infirmary creeps into the workhouse, or the sternness of workhouse rules cripples the benevolent energy which should rule the infirmary. And the treatment of the able-bodied pauper becomes too lax, or he is tempted to scheme, and does scheme, to get himself transferred to the more comfortable quarters close at hand; a desire so prevalent as to give rise to malingering—the wilful production of disease: while, partly no doubt in order to counteract this tendency, there is in such mixed establishments an unconscious disposition to treat the hospital patient with the same stern economy that is justly made the rule in dealing with able-bodied pauperism, but which, in the infirmary, is not only cruel, but in the long run is not truly economical. Another most serious evil is entailed upon the hospital by connexion with the workhouse. The habits and traditions prevalent among the habitual paupers—able-bodied paupers—in the workhouse (at least in the workhouse of a large town), are too often deeply infected with cunning, deception, and dishonesty of all sorts, against which strict precaution and stern repression are requisite; and it is most important that no communication should be allowed, whereby these habits of vice and stratagem might be introduced into the hospital, where indulgence is the rule, and where many things strictly denied to the inmates of the workhouse, as stimulants for instance, are necessarily permitted. The introduction of workhouse tricks into a hospital, where they cannot be met by workhouse control, must bring in an element of confusion, disorder, and waste, and therefore the intercommunication which might introduce those tricks should be as effectually prevented as possible, which it cannot be while the two institutions are, as at present, combined. The two systems—to use an English word in its French sense—demoralize each other; and even in the English sense, their union demoralizes the individuals subject to each.

When this is better understood and more clearly apprehended, as it soon will be, through the experience of several Unions in which the separation has been already resolved on—it is probable that it will be enforced by law. This may be expected to take place in no very long time; and then it will be found that any expenditure incurred in providing increased accommodation on a plan which does not recognise the necessity of separation has been, in part at least, thrown away; and the work will have to be done, and the money to be spent, over again.

1.Jump up ↑ Liverpool is a seaport, and a receptacle where the poverty and vice of Great Britain and Ireland seem to accumulate; and it is probably on this account that the able-bodied female paupers are peculiarly vicious and worthless.

2.Jump up ↑ Among the replies of the London medical officers, one which seemed especially to impress the Sub-Committee was given by the senior honorary medical officer of St. Thomas's. Mr. Hagger asked him, "If you had to cure the sick by contract at so much a head, and had to choose between unpaid pauper nurses allotted to you gratis, or paying yourself for skilled nurses, which would you choose?" "To pay for skilled nurses, certainly," was the unhesitating answer.

3.Jump up ↑ In the opinion of the medical men of the Liverpool Workhouse Hospital, 647 of its present number of patients would be admissible to an ordinary and n a training school for superior nurses, it will never be desirable to employ pauper under-nurses, as they interfere with the efficiency of the probationers, who are being trained as superior nurses. The latter are apt to delegate to the paupers much of the hard but most instructive part of their work. In ordinary workhouse hospitals, when there are no probationers, a certain number of pauper assistants may perhaps be useful in aiding thoroughly trained nurses.

Florence Nightingale

Florence Nightingale, OM, RRC (12 May 1820 – 13 August 1910) was a celebrated English social reformer and statistician, and the founder of modern nursing.

She came to prominence while serving as a manager of nurses trained by her during the Crimean War, where she organised the tending to wounded soldiers.[1] She gave nursing a highly favourable reputation and became an icon of Victorian culture, especially in the persona of "The Lady with the Lamp" making rounds of wounded soldiers at night.[2]

Some recent commentators have asserted Nightingale's achievements in the Crimean War were exaggerated by the media at the time, to satisfy the public's need for a hero. Nevertheless, critics agree on the decisive importance of her follow-up achievements in professionalising nursing roles for women. In 1860, Nightingale laid the foundation of professional nursing with the establishment of her nursing school at St Thomas' Hospital in London. It was the first secular nursing school in the world, now part of King's College London. The Nightingale Pledge taken by new nurses was named in her honour, and the annual International Nurses Day is celebrated around the world on her birthday. Her social reforms include improving healthcare for all sections of British society, advocating better hunger relief in India, helping to abolish prostitution laws that were over-harsh to women, and expanding the acceptable forms of female participation in the workforce.

Nightingale was a prodigious and versatile writer. In her lifetime, much of her published work was concerned with spreading medical knowledge. Some of her tracts were written in simple English so that they could easily be understood by those with poor literary skills. She also helped popularise the graphical presentation of statistical data. Much of her writing, including her extensive work on religion and mysticism, has only been published posthumously.

Early life

Florence Nightingale was born on 12 May 1820 into a rich, upper-class, well-connected British family at the Villa Colombaia,[3] in Florence, Italy, and was named after the city of her birth. Florence's older sister Frances Parthenope had similarly been named after her place of birth, Parthenope, a Greek settlement now part of the city of Naples. The family moved back to England in 1821, with Nightingale being brought up in the family's homes at Embley, Hampshire and Lea Hurst, Derbyshire.[4][5]

Her parents were William Edward Nightingale, born William Edward Shore (1794–1874) and Frances ("Fanny") Nightingale née Smith (1789–1880). William's mother Mary née Evans was the niece of Peter Nightingale, under the terms of whose will William inherited his estate at Lea Hurst, and assumed the name and arms of Nightingale. Fanny's father (Florence's maternal grandfather) was the abolitionist and Unitarian William Smith.[6] Nightingale's father educated her.[5]

In 1838, her father took the family on a tour in Europe where he was introduced to the English-born Parisian hostess Mary Clarke. Florence bonded with this woman. She recorded that "Clarkey" was a stimulating hostess who did not care for her appearance but although her idea might not always agree with her guests but "she was incapable of boring anyone." Her behaviour was said to be exasperating and eccentric and she had no respect for upper-class British women, whom she regarded generally as inconsequential. She said that if given the choice between being a woman or a galley slave, then she would choose the freedom of the galleys. She generally rejected female company and spent her time with male intellectuals. However, Clarkey made an exception in the case of the Nightingale family and Florence in particular. She and Florence were to remain close friends for 40 years despite their 27-year age difference. Clarke demonstrated that women could be equals to men, an idea that Florence had not obtained from her mother.[7]

Nightingale underwent the first of several experiences that she believed were calls from God in February 1837 while at Embley Park, prompting a strong desire to devote her life to the service of others. In her youth she was respectful of her family's opposition to her working as a nurse, only announcing her decision to enter the field in 1844. Despite the intense anger and distress of her mother and sister, she rebelled against the expected role for a woman of her status to become a wife and mother. Nightingale worked hard to educate herself in the art and science of nursing, in the face of opposition from her family and the restrictive social code for affluent young English women.[8]

As a young woman, Nightingale was attractive, slender and graceful. While her demeanour was often severe, she could be very charming and her smile was radiant. Her most persistent suitor was the politician and poet Richard Monckton Milnes, but after a nine-year courtship she rejected him, convinced that marriage would interfere with her ability to follow her calling to nursing.[8]

In Rome in 1847, she met Sidney Herbert, a politician who had been Secretary at War (1845–1846) who was on his honeymoon. He and Nightingale became lifelong close friends. Herbert would be Secretary of War again during the Crimean War, when he and his wife would be instrumental in facilitating Nightingale's nursing work in the Crimea. She became Herbert's key adviser throughout his political career, though she was accused by some of having hastened Herbert's death from Bright's Disease in 1861 because of the pressure her programme of reform placed on him.

Nightingale also much later had strong relations with academic Benjamin Jowett, who may have wanted to marry her.

Nightingale continued her travels (now with Charles and Selina Bracebridge) as far as Greece and Egypt. Her writings on Egypt in particular are testimony to her learning, literary skill and philosophy of life. Sailing up the Nile as far as Abu Simbel in January 1850, she wrote of the Abu Simbel temples, "Sublime in the highest style of intellectual beauty, intellect without effort, without suffering ... not a feature is correct—but the whole effect is more expressive of spiritual grandeur than anything I could have imagined. It makes the impression upon one that thousands of voices do, uniting in one unanimous simultaneous feeling of enthusiasm or emotion, which is said to overcome the strongest man."[9]

At Thebes, she wrote of being "called to God," while a week later near Cairo she wrote in her diary (as distinct from her far longer letters that her elder sister Parthenope was to print after her return): "God called me in the morning and asked me would I do good for him alone without reputation."[9] Later in 1850, she visited the Lutheran religious community at Kaiserswerth-am-Rhein in Germany, where she observed Pastor Theodor Fliedner and the deaconesses working for the sick and the deprived. She regarded the experience as a turning point in her life, and issued her findings anonymously in 1851; The Institution of Kaiserswerth on the Rhine, for the Practical Training of Deaconesses, etc. was her first published work.[10] She also received four months of medical training at the institute, which formed the basis for her later care.

On 22 August 1853, Nightingale took the post of superintendent at the Institute for the Care of Sick Gentlewomen in Upper Harley Street, London, a position she held until October 1854.[11] Her father had given her an annual income of £500 (roughly £40,000/US$65,000 in present terms), which allowed her to live comfortably and to pursue her career.

Crimean War

Florence Nightingale's most famous contribution came during the Crimean War, which became her central focus when reports got back to Britain about the horrific conditions for the wounded. On 21 October 1854, she and the staff of 38 women volunteer nurses that she trained, including her aunt Mai Smith,[12] and 15 Catholic nuns (mobilised by Henry Edward Manning)[13] were sent (under the authorisation of Sidney Herbert) to the Ottoman Empire. Nightingale was assisted in Paris by her friend Mary Clarke.[14] They were deployed about 295 nautical miles (546 km; 339 mi) across the Black Sea from

Balaklava in the Crimea, where the main British camp was based.

Nightingale arrived early in November 1854 at Selimiye Barracks in Scutari (modern-day Üsküdar in Istanbul). Her team found that poor care for wounded soldiers was being delivered by overworked medical staff in the face of official indifference. Medicines were in short supply, hygiene was being neglected, and mass infections were common, many of them fatal. There was no equipment to process food for the patients.

After Nightingale sent a plea to The Times for a government solution to the poor condition of the facilities, the British Government commissioned Isambard Kingdom Brunel to design a prefabricated hospital that could be built in England and shipped to the Dardanelles. The result was Renkioi Hospital, a civilian facility that, under the management of Dr Edmund Alexander Parkes, had a death rate less than 1/10th that of Scutari.[15]

Stephen Paget in the Dictionary of National Biography asserted that Nightingale reduced the death rate from 42% to 2%, either by making improvements in hygiene herself, or by calling for the Sanitary Commission.[16] For example, Nightingale implemented handwashing and other hygiene practices in the war hospital in which she worked.[17]

During her first winter at Scutari, 4,077 soldiers died there. Ten times more soldiers died from illnesses such as typhus, typhoid, cholera and dysentery than from battle wounds. With overcrowding, defective sewers and lack of ventilation, the Sanitary Commission had to be sent out by the British government to Scutari in March 1855, almost six months after Nightingale had arrived. The commission flushed out the sewers and improved ventilation.[18] Death rates were sharply reduced, but she never claimed credit for helping to reduce the death rate.[19] In 2001 and 2008 the BBC released documentaries that were critical of Nightingale's performance in the Crimean War, as were some follow-up articles published in The Guardian and the Sunday Times. Nightingale scholar Lynn McDonald has dismissed these criticisms as "often preposterous", arguing they are not supported by the primary sources.[5]

Nightingale still believed that the death rates were due to poor nutrition, lack of supplies, stale air and overworking of the soldiers. After she returned to Britain and began collecting evidence before the Royal Commission on the Health of the Army, she came to believe that most of the soldiers at the hospital were killed by poor living conditions. This experience influenced her later career, when she advocated sanitary living conditions as of great importance. Consequently, she reduced peacetime deaths in the army and turned her attention to the sanitary design of hospitals and the introduction of sanitation in working-class homes (see Statistics and Sanitary Reform, below).

The Lady with the Lamp

She is a "ministering angel" without any exaggeration in these hospitals, and as her slender form glides quietly along each corridor, every poor fellow's face softens with gratitude at the sight of her. When all the medical officers have retired for the night and silence and darkness have settled down upon those miles of prostrate sick, she may be observed alone, with a little lamp in her hand, making her solitary rounds.[20]

In the Crimea on 29 November 1855, the Nightingale Fund was established for the training of nurses during a public meeting to recognise Nightingale for her work in the war. There was an outpouring of generous donations. Sidney Herbert served as honorary secretary of the fund and the Duke of Cambridge was chairman. Nightingale was considered a pioneer in the concept of medical tourism as well, based on her 1856 letters describing spas in the Ottoman Empire. She detailed the health conditions, physical descriptions, dietary information, and other vital details of patients whom she directed there. The treatment there was significantly less expensive than in Switzerland.

Nightingale had £45,000 at her disposal from the Nightingale Fund to set up the Nightingale Training School at St. Thomas' Hospital on 9 July 1860. The first trained Nightingale nurses began work on 16 May 1865 at the Liverpool Workhouse Infirmary. Now called the Florence Nightingale School of Nursing and Midwifery, the school is part of King's College London. She also campaigned and raised funds for the Royal Buckinghamshire Hospital in Aylesbury near her sister's home, Claydon House.

Nightingale wrote Notes on Nursing (1859). The book served as the cornerstone of the curriculum at the Nightingale School and other nursing schools, though it was written specifically for the education of those nursing at home. Nightingale wrote "Every day sanitary knowledge, or the knowledge of nursing, or in other words, of how to put the constitution in such a state as that it will have no disease, or that it can recover from disease, takes a higher place. It is recognised as the knowledge which every one ought to have – distinct from medical knowledge, which only a profession can have".[22]

Notes on Nursing also sold well to the general reading public and is considered a classic introduction to nursing. Nightingale spent the rest of her life promoting and organising the nursing profession. In the introduction to the 1974 edition, Joan Quixley of the Nightingale School of Nursing wrote: "The book was the first of its kind ever to be written. It appeared at a time when the simple rules of health were only beginning to be known, when its topics were of vital importance not only for the well-being and recovery of patients, when hospitals were riddled with infection, when nurses were still mainly regarded as ignorant, uneducated persons. The book has, inevitably, its place in the history of nursing, for it was written by the founder of modern nursing".[23]

As Mark Bostridge has recently demonstrated, one of Nightingale's signal achievements was the introduction of trained nurses into the workhouse system in England and Ireland from the 1860s onwards. This meant that sick paupers were no longer being cared for by other, able-bodied paupers, but by properly trained nursing staff.

Though Nightingale is sometimes said to have denied the theory of infection for her entire life, a recent biography disagrees,[24] saying that she was simply opposed to a precursor of germ theory known as contagionism. This theory held that diseases could only be transmitted by touch. Before the experiments of the mid-1860s by Pasteur and Lister, hardly anyone took germ theory seriously; even afterwards, many medical practitioners were unconvinced. Bostridge points out that in the early 1880s Nightingale wrote an article for a textbook in which she advocated strict precautions designed, she said, to kill germs. Nightingale's work served as an inspiration for nurses in the American Civil War. The Union government approached her for advice in organising field medicine. Although her ideas met official resistance, they inspired the volunteer body of the United States Sanitary Commission.

In the 1870s, Nightingale mentored Linda Richards, "America's first trained nurse", and enabled her to return to the USA with adequate training and knowledge to establish high-quality nursing schools. Richards went on to become a nursing pioneer in the USA and Japan.

By 1882, several Nightingale nurses had become matrons at several leading hospitals, including, in London (St Mary's Hospital, Westminster Hospital, St Marylebone Workhouse Infirmary and the Hospital for Incurables at Putney) and throughout Britain (Royal Victoria Hospital, Netley; Edinburgh Royal Infirmary; Cumberland Infirmary and Liverpool Royal Infirmary), as well as at Sydney Hospital in New South Wales, Australia.

In 1883, Nightingale was awarded the Royal Red Cross by Queen Victoria. In 1904, she was appointed a Lady of Grace of the Order of St John (LGStJ). In 1907, she became the first woman to be awarded the Order of Merit. In the following year she was given the Honorary Freedom of the City of London. Her birthday is now celebrated as International CFS Awareness Day.[25]

From 1857 onwards, Nightingale was intermittently bedridden and suffered from depression. A recent biography cites brucellosis and associated spondylitis as the cause.[26] Most authorities today accept that Nightingale suffered from a particularly extreme form of brucellosis, the effects of which only began to lift in the early 1880s. Despite her symptoms, she remained phenomenally productive in social reform. During her bedridden years, she also did pioneering work in the field of hospital planning, and her work propagated quickly across Britain and the world. Nightingale's output slowed down considerably in her last decade. She wrote very little during that period due to blindness and declining mental abilities, though she still retained an interest in current affairs.[5]

Relationships

Although much of Nightingale's work improved the lot of women everywhere, Nightingale was of the opinion that women craved sympathy and were not as capable as men.[27] She criticised early women's rights activists for decrying an alleged lack of careers for women at the same time that lucrative medical positions, under the supervision of Nightingale and others, went perpetually unfilled.[28] She preferred the friendship of powerful men, insisting they had done more than women to help her attain her goals, writing: "I have never found one woman who has altered her life by one iota for me or my opinions."[29][30] She often referred to herself in the masculine, as for example "a man of action" and "a man of business".[31]

However, she did have several important and long-lasting friendships with women. Later in life, she kept up a prolonged correspondence with Irish nun Sister Mary Clare Moore, with whom she had worked in Crimea.[32] Her most beloved confidante was Mary Clarke, an Englishwoman she met in 1837 and kept in touch with throughout her life.[33]

Some scholars of Nightingale's life believe that she remained chaste for her entire life, perhaps because she felt a religious calling to her career.[34]

Death

On 13 August 1910, at the age of 90, she died peacefully in her sleep in her room at 10 South Street, Mayfair, London.[35][36] The offer of burial in Westminster Abbey was declined by her relatives and she is buried in the graveyard at St Margaret's Church in East Wellow, Hampshire, near Embley Park.[37][38] She left a large body of work, including several hundred notes that were previously unpublished.[39] A memorial monument to Nightingale was created in Carrara marble by Francis William Sargant in 1913 and placed in the cloister of the Basilica of Santa Croce, Florence.[40]

Contributions

Florence Nightingale exhibited a gift for mathematics from an early age and excelled in the subject under the tutorship of her father.[41] Later, Nightingale became a pioneer in the visual presentation of information and statistical graphics.[42] She used methods such as the pie chart, which had first been developed by William Playfair in 1801. While taken for granted now, it was at the time a relatively novel method of presenting data.[43]

Indeed, Nightingale is described as "a true pioneer in the graphical representation of statistics", and is credited with developing a form of the pie chart now known as the polar area diagram,[44] or occasionally the Nightingale rose diagram, equivalent to a modern circular histogram, to illustrate seasonal sources of patient mortality in the military field hospital she managed. Nightingale called a compilation of such diagrams a "coxcomb", but later that term would frequently be used for the individual diagrams.[45] She made extensive use of coxcombs to present reports on the nature and magnitude of the conditions of medical care in the Crimean War to Members of Parliament and civil servants who would have been unlikely to read or understand traditional statistical reports. In 1859, Nightingale was elected the first female member of the Royal Statistical Society. She later became an honorary member of the American Statistical Association.

Her attention turned to the health of the British army in India and she demonstrated that bad drainage, contaminated water, overcrowding and poor ventilation were causing the high death rate. She concluded that the health of the army and the people of India had to go hand in hand and so campaigned to improve the sanitary conditions of the country as a whole.

Nightingale made a comprehensive statistical study of sanitation in Indian rural life and was the leading figure in the introduction of improved medical care and public health service in India. In 1858 and 1859, she successfully lobbied for the establishment of a Royal Commission into the Indian situation. Two years later, she provided a report to the commission, which completed its own study in 1863. "After 10 years of sanitary reform, in 1873, Nightingale reported that mortality among the soldiers in India had declined from 69 to 18 per 1,000".[44]

The Royal Sanitary Commission of 1868–9 presented Nightingale with an opportunity to press for compulsory sanitation in private houses. She lobbied the minister responsible, James Stansfeld, to strengthen the proposed Public Health Bill to require owners of existing properties to pay for connection to mains drainage.[46] The strengthened legislation was enacted in the Public Health Acts of 1874 and 1875. At the same time she combined with the retired sanitary reformer Edwin Chadwick to persuade Stansfeld to devolve powers to enforce the law to Local Authorities, eliminating central control by medical technocrats.[47] Her Crimean War statistics had convinced her that non-medical approaches were more effective given the state of knowledge at the time. Historians now believe that both drainage and devolved enforcement played a crucial role in increasing average national life expectancy by 20 years between 1871 and the mid-1930s during which time medical science made no impact on the most fatal epidemic diseases.[19][48]

Literature and the women's movement

" Nightingale's achievements are all the more impressive when they are considered against the background of social restraints on women in Victorian England. Her father, William Edward Nightingale, was an extremely wealthy landowner, and the family moved in the highest circles of English society. In those days, women of Nightingale's class did not attend universities and did not pursue professional careers; their purpose in life was to marry and bear children. Nightingale was fortunate. Her father believed women should be educated, and he personally taught her Italian, Latin, Greek, philosophy, history and – most unusual of all for women of the time – writing and mathematics.[49] "

While better known for her contributions in the nursing and mathematical fields, Nightingale is also an important link in the study of English feminism. During 1850 and 1852, she was struggling with her self-definition and the expectations of an upper-class marriage from her family. As she sorted out her thoughts, she wrote Suggestions for Thought to Searchers after Religious Truth. This was an 829-page, three-volume work, which Nightingale had printed privately in 1860, but which until recently was never published in its entirety.[50] An effort to correct this was made with a 2008 publication by Wilfrid Laurier University, as volume 11[51] of a 16 volume project, the Collected Works of Florence Nightingale.[52] The best known of these essays, called "Cassandra", was previously published by Ray Strachey in 1928. Strachey included it in The Cause, a history of the women's movement. Apparently, the writing served its original purpose of sorting out thoughts; Nightingale left soon after to train at the Institute for deaconesses at Kaiserswerth.

"Cassandra" protests the over-feminisation of women into near helplessness, such as Nightingale saw in her mother's and older sister's lethargic lifestyle, despite their education. She rejected their life of thoughtless comfort for the world of social service. The work also reflects her fear of her ideas being ineffective, as were Cassandra's. Cassandra was a princess of Troy who served as a priestess in the temple of Apollo during the Trojan War. The god gave her the gift of prophecy; when she refused his advances, he cursed her so that her prophetic warnings would go unheeded. Elaine Showalter called Nightingale's writing "a major text of English feminism, a link between Wollstonecraft and Woolf."[53]

Theology

Despite being named as a Unitarian in several older sources, Nightingale's own rare references to conventional Unitarianism are mildly negative. She remained in the Church of England throughout her life, albeit with unorthodox views. Influenced from an early age by the Wesleyan tradition, Nightingale felt that genuine religion should manifest in active care and love for others.[54][55] She wrote a work of theology: Suggestions for Thought, her own theodicy, which develops her heterodox ideas. Nightingale questioned the goodness of a God who would condemn souls to hell, and was a believer in universal reconciliation – the concept that even those who die without being saved will eventually make it to Heaven.[56] She would sometimes comfort those in her care with this view. For example, a dying young prostitute being tended by Nightingale was concerned she was going to hell and said to her 'Pray God, that you may never be in the despair I am in at this time'. The nurse replied "Oh, my girl, are you not now more merciful than the God you think you are going to? Yet the real God is far more merciful than any human creature ever was or can ever imagine."[4][30][57][58]

Despite her intense personal devotion to Christ, Nightingale believed for much of her life that the pagan and eastern religions had also contained genuine revelation. She was a strong opponent of discrimination both against Christians of different denominations, and against those of non-Christian religions. Nightingale believed religion helped provide people with the fortitude for arduous good work, and would ensure the nurses in her care attended religious services. However she was often critical of organised religion. She disliked the role the 19th century Church of England would sometimes play in worsening the oppression of the poor. Nightingale argued that secular hospitals usually provided better care than their religious counterparts. While she held that the ideal health professional should be inspired by a religious as well as professional motive, she said that in practice many religiously motivated health workers were concerned chiefly in securing their own salvation, and that this motivation was inferior to the professional desire to deliver the best possible care.[4][30]

Legacy

Nightingale's lasting contribution has been her role in founding the modern nursing profession. She set an example of compassion, commitment to patient care and diligent and thoughtful hospital administration. The first official nurses' training programme, her Nightingale School for Nurses, opened in 1860. In addition to the continued operation of the Florence Nightingale School of Nursing and Midwifery at King's College London, the Nightingale Building in the School of Nursing and Midwifery at the University of Southampton is also named after her.

In 1912, the International Committee of the Red Cross instituted the Florence Nightingale Medal, awarded every two years to nurses or nursing aides for outstanding service. Since 1965, International Nurses Day has been celebrated on her birthday each year. The President of India honours nursing professionals with the "National Florence Nightingale Award" every year on International Nurses Day. The award, established in 1973, is given in recognition of meritorious services of nursing professionals characterised by devotion, sincerity, dedication and compassion.

The Florence Nightingale Declaration Campaign,[59] established by nursing leaders throughout the world through the Nightingale Initiative for Global Health (NIGH), aims to build a global grassroots movement to achieve two United Nations Resolutions for adoption by the UN General Assembly of 2008. They will declare: The International Year of the Nurse–2010 (the centennial of Nightingale's death); The UN Decade for a Healthy World–2011 to 2020 (the bicentennial of Nightingale's birth). NIGH also works to rekindle awareness about the important issues highlighted by Florence Nightingale, such as preventive medicine and holistic health. So far, the Florence Nightingale Declaration has been signed by over 18,500 signatories from 86 countries.

During the Vietnam War, Nightingale inspired many US Army nurses, sparking a renewal of interest in her life and work. Her admirers include Country Joe of Country Joe and the Fish, who has assembled an extensive website in her honour.[60]

The Agostino Gemelli Medical School[61] in Rome, the first university-based hospital in Italy and one of its most respected medical centres, honoured Nightingale's contribution to the nursing profession by giving the name "Bedside Florence" to a wireless computer system it developed to assist nursing.[62]

Hospitals

Four hospitals in Istanbul are named after Nightingale: Florence Nightingale Hospital in Şişli (the biggest private hospital in Turkey), Metropolitan Florence Nightingale Hospital in Gayrettepe, European Florence Nightingale Hospital in Mecidiyeköy, and Kızıltoprak Florence Nightingale Hospital in Kadiköy, all belonging to the Turkish Cardiology Foundation.[63]

An appeal is being considered for the former Derbyshire Royal Infirmary hospital in Derby, England to be named after Nightingale. The suggested new name will be either Nightingale Community Hospital or Florence Nightingale Community Hospital. The area in which the hospital lies in Derby has recently been referred to as the "Nightingale Quarter".[64]

Museums and monuments

Statue of Florence Nightingale in Waterloo Place, London

There are three statues of Nightingale in Derby – one outside the London Road Community Hospital formerly known as the Derbyshire Royal Infirmary (DRI), one in St Peter's Street, and one above the Nightingale-Macmillan Continuing Care Unit opposite the Derbyshire Royal Infirmary. A public house named after her stands close to the DRI.[65] The Nightingale-Macmillan continuing care unit is now at the Royal Derby Hospital, formerly known as The City Hospital, Derby.

A stained glass window was commissioned for inclusion in the Derbyshire Royal Infirmary chapel in the late 1950s. When the chapel was demolished the window was removed and installed in the replacement chapel. At the closure of the DRI the window was again removed and stored. In October 2010, £6,000 was raised to reposition the window in St Peter's Church, Derby. The work features nine panels, of the original ten, depicting scenes of hospital life, Derby townscapes and Nightingale herself. Some of the work was damaged and the tenth panel was dismantled for the glass to be used in repair of the remaining panels. All the figures, who are said to be modelled on prominent Derby town figures of the early sixties, surround and praise a central pane of the triumphant Christ. A nurse who posed for the top right panel in 1959 attended the rededication service in October 2010.[66]

The Florence Nightingale Museum at St Thomas' Hospital in London reopened in May 2010 in time for the centenary of Nightingale's death. Another museum devoted to her is at her sister's family home, Claydon House, now a property of the National Trust.

Upon the centenary of Nightingale's death in 2010, and to commemorate her connection with Malvern, the Malvern Museum held a Florence Nightingale exhibit[67] with a school poster competition to promote some events.[68]

In Istanbul, the northernmost tower of the Selimiye Barracks building is now the Florence Nightingale Museum.[69] and in several of its rooms, relics and reproductions related to Florence Nightingale and her nurses are on exhibition.[70]

When Nightingale moved on to the Crimea itself in May 1855, she often travelled on horseback to make hospital inspections. She later transferred to a mule cart and was reported to have escaped serious injury when the cart was toppled in an accident. Following this, she used a solid Russian-built carriage, with a waterproof hood and curtains. The carriage was returned to England by Alexis Soyer after the war and subsequently given to the Nightingale training school. The carriage was damaged when the hospital was bombed during the Second World War. It was restored and transferred to the Army Medical Services Museum, now in Mytchett, Surrey, near Aldershot.

A bronze plaque, attached to the plinth of the Crimean Memorial in the Haydarpaşa Cemetery, Istanbul and unveiled on Empire Day, 1954, to celebrate the 100th anniversary of her nursing service in that region, bears the inscription: "To Florence Nightingale, whose work near this Cemetery a century ago relieved much human suffering and laid the foundations for the nursing profession."[71]

Audio

Florence Nightingale's voice was saved for posterity in a phonograph recording from 1890 preserved in the British Library Sound Archive. The recording, made in aid of the Light Brigade Relief Fund and available to hear online, says:

When I am no longer even a memory, just a name, I hope my voice may perpetuate the great work of my life. God bless my dear old comrades of Balaclava and bring them safe to shore. Florence Nightingale.[72]

Theatre

The first theatrical representation of Nightingale was Reginald Berkeley's The Lady with the Lamp, premiering in London in 1929 with Edith Evans in the title role. It did not portray her as an entirely sympathetic character and draws much characterisation from Lytton Strachey's biography of her in Eminent Victorians.[73] It was adapted as a film of the same name in 1951.

In 2009, a stage musical play representation of Nightingale entitled The Voyage of the Lass was produced by the Association of Nursing Service Administrators of the Philippines. The play tells the story of Nightingale's early life and her struggles during the Crimean War, showcasing Philippine local registered nurses from various hospitals of the country.[citation needed]

Film

In 1912, a biographical silent film titled The Victoria Cross, starring Julia Swayne Gordon as Nightingale, was released, followed in 1915 by another silent film, Florence Nightingale, featuring Elisabeth Risdon. In 1936, Kay Francis played Nightingale in the film titled The White Angel. In 1951, The Lady With the Lamp starred Anna Neagle.

Television

Portrayals of Nightingale on television, in documentary as in fiction, vary – the BBC's 2008 Florence Nightingale emphasised her independence and feeling of religious calling, but in Channel 4's 2006 Mary Seacole: The Real Angel of the Crimea she is portrayed as narrow-minded and opposed to Seacole's efforts. In 1985, a TV biopic Florence Nightingale, starring Jaclyn Smith, was produced.[74]

Banknotes

Florence Nightingale's image appeared on the reverse of £10 Series D banknotes issued by the Bank of England from 1975 until 1994. As well as a standing portrait, she was depicted on the notes in a field hospital, holding her lamp.[75]

Photographs

Nightingale had a principled objection to having photographs taken or her portrait painted. An extremely rare photograph of her, taken at Embley on a visit to her family home in May 1858, was discovered in 2006 and is now at the Florence Nightingale Museum in London. A black-and-white photograph taken in about 1907 by Lizzie Caswall Smith at Nightingale's London home in South Street, Park Lane, was auctioned on 19 November 2008 by Dreweatts auction house in Newbury, Berkshire, England, for £5,500.[76]

Biographies

The first biography of Nightingale was published in England in 1855. In 1911, Edward Tyas Cook was authorised by Nightingale's executors to write the official life, published in two volumes in 1913. Lytton Strachey based much of his chapter on Nightingale in Eminent Victorians on Cook, and Cecil Woodham-Smith also relied heavily on Cook's Life in her 1950 biography, though she did have access to new family material preserved at Claydon. In 2008, Mark Bostridge published a major new life of Nightingale, almost exclusively based on unpublished material from the Verney Collections at Claydon and from archival documents from about 200 archives around the world, some of which had been published by Lynn McDonald in her projected sixteen-volume edition of the Collected Works of Florence Nightingale (2001 to date).

www.ingramcontent.com/pod-product-compliance
Lightning Source LLC
Chambersburg PA
CBHW070335190526
45169CB00005B/1909